THE POST-LSD SYNDROME

Diagnosis and Treatment
Revised Edition

Edwin I. Roth, M.D.

authorHOUSE®

AuthorHouse™
1663 Liberty Drive
Bloomington, IN 47403
www.authorhouse.com
Phone: 1 (800) 839-8640

© *2018 Edwin I. Roth, M.D. All rights reserved.*

No part of this book may be reproduced, stored in a retrieval system, or transmitted by any means without the written permission of the author.

Published by AuthorHouse 07/06/2018

ISBN: 978-1-5462-4475-2 (sc)
ISBN: 978-1-5462-4474-5 (e)

Library of Congress Control Number: 2018906971

Print information available on the last page.

Any people depicted in stock imagery provided by Getty Images are models, and such images are being used for illustrative purposes only. Certain stock imagery © Getty Images.

This book is printed on acid-free paper.

Because of the dynamic nature of the Internet, any web addresses or links contained in this book may have changed since publication and may no longer be valid. The views expressed in this work are solely those of the author and do not necessarily reflect the views of the publisher, and the publisher hereby disclaims any responsibility for them.

Contents

Dedication vii
Foreword ix

Chapter 1 The Clinical Syndrome 1
Chapter 2 LSD 15
Chapter 3 Treatment, Course of Illness,
           and Prognosis 23
Chapter 4 Alcoholism 31
Chapter 5 Depression 37
Chapter 6 Addiction 40
Chapter 7 Suicide 43
Chapter 8 Special Cases 47
Chapter 9 Barry 54

Bibliography 59
Author Biography 61

DEDICATION

To Physicians,
And to the Patients they Serve

Foreword

After more than 30 years of private and institutional practice of Psychiatry and Psychoanalysis in Ohio, health issues dictated I move to southern California in 1997. Working with out-patients in my private practice and in a County Clinic, and then with inmates in a State prison, I gradually realized that five to ten per cent of the patients I was encountering represented a group of patients I had not recognized or heard of before, and diagnosed more than 300 patients with THE POST-LSD SYNDROME. These patients were acutely and severely ill, yet surprisingly, I found nothing in the literature describing their condition, which led me to write my previous book on this subject.

In the ensuing years, I have continued my private practice and also became the Treating Psychiatrist on a Psychiatric unit, thereby gaining experience with a more impaired set of patients. The occurrence rate has been consistent, and I have now treated about 500 patients. The additional data provided by patients and time to reflect on all the data have led to some important changes in my understanding of this condition. I have incorporated these revisions into this book and hope this will be helpful in providing effective treatment for these patients.

Chapter 1

The Clinical Syndrome

I want to bring attention to a generally unrecognized, serious, at times severe, dysfunction in people, which is usually misdiagnosed as an emotional problem, but is actually an organic disturbance of brain function caused by the prolonged effect of LSD. I have termed this condition The Post-LSD Syndrome. The bad news is that there is a severe condition, The Post-LSD Syndrome (TPLSDS), which can result from even a single exposure to LSD, even decades after the exposure. The good news is that proper treatment can induce a complete remission fairly easily.

As I see it, TPLSDS is a discrete, unique group of severe symptoms which can be viewed as a tetrad of 1) a severe anxiety state, 2) a severe sleep disturbance, 3) impaired intellectual functioning, and 4) emotional instability. Most patients experience an acute onset with extreme anxiety, panic, inability to sleep, inability to concentrate and think clearly, and surges of emotion. Some fear they are becoming psychotic. Many patients remain acutely symptomatic for years unless treated effectively. Among the patients I saw, none had received effective treatment, and had been ill for months or years. Some had gone into a spontaneous remission for a time, then had a recurrence of symptoms. This cycle can occur repeatedly. Some patients who are acutely ill for a prolonged period may eventually go into a chronic phase which I will discuss below.

The Symptoms of the Basic Condition

The following is a detailed description of the symptoms and clinical findings of the tetrad that constitutes the basic condition of the TPLSDS. The four symptoms may have a simultaneous onset, but frequently the anxiety is primary, followed within a few days by the insomnia. The impaired intellectual functioning follows in a few days to several weeks, and the emotional instability accompanies it, or follows shortly after. By the time a physician is consulted, usually all symptoms are present.

1) The anxiety is a severe and most distressing symptom, often close to a panic state, and usually causes patients to seek treatment. They usually have no psychological explanation for their anxiety. This overwhelming anxiety is often accompanied

by a sense of dread, doom, and despair and a fear of impending death. It is akin to what was termed LSD panic in the past. It can occur frequently, last for hours, and even be present most of the time, interfering severely with ability to function. Some patients say they would rather be dead than experience the severe anxiety for a prolonged period.

The anxiety often causes somatic symptoms, e.g., dyspnea, tachycardia, chest pain, weakness, sweating, dizziness, and faintness. Patients often present at an Emergency Room fearing a heart attack, and some have been briefly admitted to a Cardiac Unit. This severe anxiety causes patients to desperately seek a measure of relief, and they turn to medications, alcohol, or illegal drugs with incomplete benefit, but many become addicted while seeking relief.

Some patients linked their feeling of panic to prior experience with LSD, and said they experienced the same panic currently as they did when they used LSD months or years previously. Some reported reexperiencing somatic symptoms; e.g., visual distortions, hallucinations, odors, a bad taste, etc. One patient reported a sequence of tightening of his throat, then feeling unable to breathe, and then having a bad taste in his throat just as he'd experienced during his last few LSD trips many years previously. It was these connections to LSD which patients brought which enabled me to recognize the role of LSD in causing TPLSDS. Surprisingly, patients consistently reported that doctors insisted that LSD was unrelated to their condition, even when the patients told of their past use and the return of old symptoms caused by the past use.

2) The sleep disturbance, like the anxiety, is present in virtually all patients with this condition, and is equally responsible for patients seeking treatment. The sleep problem has unique, distressing qualities. It typically consists of severe insomnia, racing thoughts when trying to fall asleep, and vivid, terrifying nightmares. Patients are unable to fall asleep, tossing for hours, sleep fitfully, and awaken frequently. They achieve little or no sound sleep, and are irritable and exhausted, unable to function the next day, especially at work. They often resort to a variety of measures, particularly prescription medications, alcohol, and/or marijuana, to try to gain some sleep.

They report racing thoughts may occur during the day, but are particularly prominent at night. Patients describe thinking rapidly of one thing after another, jumping from subject to subject, with a feeling that the mind can't shut off. They feel they have no control over their thoughts, which they describe with metaphors such as a runaway train, a tornado of thoughts, and a movie that never ends. The thoughts cover all subjects which concern them, and the patients report their minds jump from one subject to another without resolving any of the concerns and without formulating any constructive course of action.

The unique, distressing nightmares are the final and most significant symptom of the sleep disturbance. They are remarkably vivid, intense, horrible, usually bizarre and unreal, and typically have a psychotic-like lack of restraint and control. The dreamer typically awakens disoriented and terrified, convinced that the dream was real, and is greatly relieved when able to gradually reorient and realize he was dreaming.

The dreams may present a realistic situation, or an actual memory, in an extreme and distorted way, or a bizarre, unreal situation involving monsters, aliens, or devils. The dreamer typically is threatened in a very dangerous situation, is often on the verge of being killed, and may even actually die in the dream, which rarely occurs in the common nightmare. Or a loved one, such as a child, may be in mortal danger, and may actually be murdered. The dreamer may kill assailants to defend the child or himself. The dreams often are in color, and bloody.

Many patients cannot fall asleep after awakening from one of these horrible dreams for fear it will recur. Many patients who do not dream actually abort the dreams by awakening frequently, and thus they may report that they sleep very little. It cannot be overemphasized how uniquely horrible, terrifying, and upsetting these dreams are, with an unusual intensity and vividness that is usually seen only in a delirium or a psychosis. I believe these dreams are pathognomonic of TPLSDS when they occur in the absence of a psychosis or a delirium.

3) The impaired intellectual functioning is mild to severe and can be devastating. Patients feel distracted and unable to focus, concentrate, or think clearly. They often are unable to watch TV or play a game. They may become unable to read, finding themselves rereading pages and unable to recall what they just read. Their memory deteriorates, and they may become unable to study, work, or learn. They become unable to think through and solve problems. Some fail academically or withdraw from classes, some quit or lose their jobs, and some fail in their businesses. However, patients retain a core of healthy ego and superego functioning, with judgement, standards, values, ambition, goals, and

relationships, and thus are distressed by their inability to function, the resultant harm to their careers, and the financial consequences to their families. They cannot explain their dysfunction and feel upset with themselves as if they are voluntarily misbehaving. On superficial examination some patients appear to be intact, as their mental status performance on general knowledge, abstractions, calculations, etc. is often adequate. However, most report they are not responding as well as they should; they feel something is blocking their mind.

4) The emotional instability is described by patients as getting stressed easily and becoming overwhelmed with emotion, usually anger or tears. Many become tearful easily and embarrass themselves by crying in public with only mild provocation. Some become irritable and argumentative, may get surges of anger which are difficult to control, and may have violent impulses which are not characteristic of them. As a result of this emotional lability, many feel uncomfortable around people and seek to withdraw and isolate themselves. Objectively, this emotional lability may be seen as tearfulness or anger in the clinical session, and the patients may feel embarrassed and apologize. In some patients, especially men

who have experienced TPLSDS for years, the anger surges may be prominent, even dominating, and lead to brawling and sadism. Such patients may feel this behavior is an inherent part of their personality which could never change. However, the anger may actually be ego-alien and undesirable, and some patients become aware that they dislike the aggression after they begin to benefit from treatment.

Let me describe some typical patients to bring the clinical picture into a clear focus. These patients demonstrate remarkable similarities in their presentation and discussion of their clinical pathology, and their response to treatment. In this section I will refer to treatment briefly and save the comprehensive discussion for Chapter Three.

Case 1) Mrs. A. was an intelligent, educated, personable 42-year old married woman who had experienced increasing anxiety and depression for two years, and sought consultation with me because she felt weekly counseling and medications were not helping. First and foremost, she had a sleep disturbance consisting of severe insomnia, racing thoughts which kept her awake for hours, and terrifying, vivid, nightmares when she finally fell asleep. She also had anxiety attacks during the day which bordered on panic and made her feel disabled and unable to function. She had trouble concentrating, and generally felt confused and distracted. An extremely competent person basicly, she knew she was performing poorly. She often felt irritable and tearful.

Her severe anxiety was prominent and impressive. She had no manifestations of psychosis, e.g., she had no thought disorder or disturbance of affect, and her ego was basically intact, although her performance and her ability to cope with anxiety, affects, and stress was impaired. She felt her satisfactory performance on the mental status exam I gave her was actually below her true ability. She denied any drug use or alcohol abuse, but, upon reflection, did recall a terrible experience at a party when she was 17. She felt something had been put into her drink because she developed a prolonged "bad trip" in which she felt panic, felt she was going to die, was frightened, agitated and paranoid, and had visual disturbances. She hallucinated and thought the walls were moving in on her. She was unable to sleep that night, but finally felt better the next day. We concluded she most likely had been slipped some LSD, which she knew was at the party. She said her mind never felt quite right after that—she always felt anxious, easily disturbed and distracted.

She agreed to medication, and I started her on a low dose of Olanzapine (Zyprexa), an antipsychotic. To her great relief and our mutual surprise, when she returned one week later she reported a remarkable improvement. Her sleep disturbance had cleared

Chapter 1

up completely! She no longer had racing thoughts, insomnia, or nightmares, and she slept soundly all night. Her anxiety had also decreased significantly. Her symptoms gradually improved over the next few weeks; she felt less distracted, more able to focus and concentrate, and was less depressed. Over the next few months her symptoms faded away. She decreased her Olanzapine, gradually discontinued her other medications, and went into full remission. She was elated and grateful, and felt she was herself again. She felt she had no need for further therapy or counseling.

Case 2) Mr. B. was a 27-year-old professional who presented severely distressed by severe anxiety, horrible nightmares, and feeling distracted and unable to focus, concentrate, or work for over a year. He was seeing a Psychiatrist who had prescribed various tranquilizers and antidepressants which did not help. He feared people could detect his anxiety, so he tried to avoid looking them in the eye and isolated himself as much as possible. His sleep was disturbed by horrible, vivid nightmares with monsters in which he was in danger, became enraged, and injured people and monsters. He dreaded these dreams, and the anger that accompanied them. He felt he stressed out easily, feared having to make a work presentation, could not cope with people or his job, cried frequently, and lost his job and his girl friend.

He felt his problems stemmed from having taken LSD two years previously, but his psychiatrists had disagreed. He said he'd had the same anxiety and inability to focus when he took the LSD hit, and then they cleared up after a few days. However, less than a year later the anxiety returned, and other symptoms started and progressed. He said he had been using a little marijuana about three times a week for years and it relaxed him. I agreed with him about the LSD and we agreed to start him on Olanzapine and to taper him off of his medications and marijuana. His symptoms improved dramatically after the first dose, and he rather quickly went into full remission. He said he felt much better with people, was ready to return to work, but first wanted to take a special trip which he and a friend had planned. He no longer felt too ill to make the trip. He said he'd take his Olanzapine at the lower dose, but hoped he could do without it soon.

Case 3) Ms. C. was an immature 21-year old woman who had been in therapy since 17 for anxiety and depression. Various medications had been unhelpful. She had just completed a one-year training program which certified her in her career, and was about to start her first job. However, a month prior to her presentation to me, she developed severe panic attacks with nausea, dizziness, difficulty breathing, insomnia, and racing thoughts. She felt unable to think clearly, and felt she was going to die. On mental status,

Chapter 1

her ego was basically intact, however, she had extreme anxiety, had trouble coping with stresses, and had trouble concentrating. She felt angry and volatile. She hoped weekly therapy would enable her to feel better and to be effective in her new job, and we agreed to start. She reduced the dosage of her antidepressant which she thought had made her worse, and reduced her use of alcohol and marijuana, which she had been taking for her insomnia. However, she then developed vividly terrifying nightmares from which she awoke in a panic.

She then revealed she had smoked some marijuana about 6 months previously which she feared had been laced with LSD, because it caused a terrifying experience in which she felt panic and nausea, couldn't breathe, and felt she was going to die. The walls felt like they were moving in on her, she saw bright colors, sounds were louder, and she felt she couldn't focus on anything. She went to an emergency room and got a shot which stopped the episode, and she thought she was over it. Her boyfriend used a lot of LSD, always pressed her to join him in using it, but had promised never to force it on her. She agreed to medication, and I prescribed Olanzapine. She immediately felt calmer after she took the first dose, and was able to sleep well. However, she felt drugged and overmedicated. We reduced the dose with excellent results. Her racing thoughts and nightmares stopped, her anxiety and anger gradually decreased, and within 3 weeks all presenting symptoms had improved considerably.

After several months she was in full remission from TPLSDS. She worked on her emotional issues in her therapy more effectively. She had much more ego strength with which to work on them, i.e., she was no longer overwhelmed by affects and anxiety because of interference from LSD effects and could gain relief from the therapeutic process. After several months she no longer felt depressed, and she decided to leave the boy friend. She continued her Olanzapine daily for over a year, gradually decreasing the dosage to every other evening, while she continued in psychotherapy for a second year until she moved out of state to go to college.

Case 4) Mr. D. was a 17-yr old high school senior who was on a holiday with his parents visiting family in my area. He had panic attacks so severe that they caused him to vomit, and he felt unable to concentrate or think. He felt he had something physically wrong and felt that he would die. He complained that for the past month he'd had insomnia, terrible nightmares, horrible rushing thoughts, and severe anxiety which culminated in the panic attacks. He felt unable to function, hadn't been able to go to school, felt agitated and irritable, ready to explode, and had recently crashed and totaled his van. He felt these symptoms were precipitated by his smoking marijuana about a month previously, because at the time he had felt weird and sick, and was reminded of a bad episode,

Chapter 1

a bad trip, he'd had about a year previously when he'd thought he had been slipped some LSD.

On mental status, he showed no signs of psychosis, but he was under great stress, and had trouble concentrating and performing intellectual tasks such as calculations and abstractions. He was extremely anxious and overwhelmed. I felt he was suffering from TPLSDS, medicated him with Olanzapine, and he responded immediately. He slept soundly the first night, and had no more rushing thoughts or nightmares. Over the next few weeks his anxiety dissipated, and he became increasingly able to concentrate, read and study. He continued his Olanzapine and was able to return home and resume school successfully.

Chapter 2

LSD

Lysergic Acid Diethylamide (LSD) has been a fascinating, seductive, dangerous, and controversial drug for decades. In 1917, Sandoz Laboratories, a Swiss pharmaceutical company, began studying ergot alkaloids, which are alkaloids produced by a fungus, ergot, which grows on grains, especially rye. In 1918 Sandoz extracted and purified ergotamine, which became a useful medication. Ergotamine causes vasoconstriction, so it has been employed to control bleeding, but it also can cause painful neuropathies and gangrene of the limbs if vasoconstriction excessively decreases blood flow. It also has neurological effects, and has been useful in treating migraine. It has strong effects on the uterine musculature, and can both stop uterine bleeding and cause the onset of labor. In Europe in the middle ages there were epidemics of ergotamine poisoning resulting from ingestion of bread made from ergot-infested rye. The epidemics caused mass

Chapter 2

illnesses and deaths. There was a gangrenous form resulting from ergotamine's vasoconstrictive effect, which was termed St. Anthony's fire. There also was a convulsive form which resulted from ergotamine's neurological effects.

In his book, Albert Hoffman described how he came to Sandoz in 1929 after completing his PhD, and in 1935 began working on ergotamine and the newly-isolated lysergic acid which was derived from it. He combined the lysergic acid with amines, and in 1938 synthesized lysergic acid diethylamide 25, LSD 25. He described setting the drug aside for 5 years, returning to it in 1943, and then experiencing an intoxication from it, which he concluded came from accidentally absorbing a small amount through his fingers. He decided to study the drug and deliberately ingested .25 mgm. He became intoxicated and experienced profound effects which he described in his book:

"The dizziness and sensation of fainting became so strong at times that I could no longer hold myself erect, and I had to lie down on the sofa. My surroundings had now transformed themselves in more terrifying ways. Everything in the room spun around, and the familiar objects and pieces of furniture assumed grotesque, threatening forms. They were in continuous motion, animated, as if driven by an inner restlessness. The lady next door, whom I scarcely recognized, brought me milk—she was a malevolent witch with a colored mask."

THE POST-LSD SYNDROME

"Even worse than these demonic transformations of the outer world, were the alterations that I perceived in myself, in my inner being. Every exertion of my will, every attempt to put an end to the disintegration of the outer world and the dissolution of my ego, seemed to be wasted effort. A demon had invaded me, had taken possession of my body, mind, and soul. I jumped up and screamed, trying to free myself from him, but then sank down again and lay helpless on the sofa. The substance, with which I had wanted to experiment, had vanquished me. It was the demon that scornfully triumphed over my will. I was seized by the dreadful fear of going insane, I was taken to another world, another place, another time. My body seemed to be without sensation, lifeless, strange. Was I dying?....

"Slowly I came back from a weird, unfamiliar world... The horror softened and gave way to a feeling of good fortune and gratitude.

"Now, little by little, I could begin to enjoy the unprecedented colors and plays of shapes that persisted behind my closed eyes."

Thus, although disconcerted and overwhelmed at first by his experience and vividly describing his perception of the "disintegration of the world and the dissolution of his ego," Hoffman twisted his experience into a positive one. He extolled the visual distortions and claimed the drug was "mind-expanding," ignoring its toxicity. He became an active, articulate proselyte for LSD, a Pied Piper who unfortunately attracted many advocates, including Alduous Huxley, Timothy Leary, and Alan Ginsburg. They organized marches and gatherings, proclaimed, "tune in, turn on, drop out" joyfully, and were oblivious of the damage they were causing in others and in themselves. Unfortunately, their efforts succeeded in helping LSD to achieve considerable popular support and use until its casualties mounted and its toxicity became so apparent that the dangers of using LSD could no longer be ignored.

In the early 1960's numerous articles were published in the press and in the Psychiatric literature describing the serious pathological consequences of using LSD., Smart and Bateman published a review article in 1967 which summarized the reports of LSD's acute toxic reactions. They reported 1) bizarre visual experiences such as heightening of brightness and color perception, distortions in the perceptions of real objects, and visual delusions or hallucinations, 2) emotional effects—apprehension, panic, elation, or depression, and 3) prolonged psychotic reactions, e.g., paranoid delusions, schizophrenic-like hallucinations, and overwhelming fear. They also reported chronic toxic reactions, namely, 4) spontaneous recurrences of parts of the LSD experience weeks or months after the last LSD ingestion and after an interval of normality, and 5) prolonged, apparently non-psychotic reactions such as acute panic, confusion, and depression. They reported that panic was the most frequent acute reaction, and its most common features were dissociation, terror, confusion, and fear of going insane and of not being able to return to normality.

There have been other reports of acute toxic reactions to LSD usage which I have included in the bibliography, a few of which I will enumerate. Ungerleider, et al, reported 70 cases of prolonged acute psychotic reactions to LSD, 68% of whom required more than one month of hospitalization. Eveloff coined the terms LSD Syndrome and LSD panic in 1968, describing LSD-caused acute ego dissolution/disintegration, which was manifested by psychotic reactions, rage, panic, and suicidal tendencies. Vardy and Kay compared acute LSD psychotic patients to first-break schizophrenics, and found them to be fundamentally similar in genealogy, phenomenology, and course of illness. Abraham and Aldridge quoted 75 cases of LSD-caused acute psychosis from 16 clinical studies, and reported the commonest symptoms were mood swings, visual hallucinations, mania, grandiosity, and religiosity. They also described Post-Hallucinogenic Perceptual Disorder (PHPD) as an adverse consequence of LSD use encompassing a variety of visual disorders. These studies, and many more, have basically described acute reactions and complications to LSD exposure, and, while long term consequences have been mentioned, there has been little documentation of significant chronic pathology.

Chapter 2

The LSD Flashback syndrome attracted considerable attention in the 1970's, and was considered to be a transient episode of recurrence of perceptual and/or emotional distortions which occurred after a period of normalcy following the use of the drug. Shick and Smith described this condition in detail, and felt it was a real and significant condition. They felt the flashbacks could last from minutes to hours, and occur from once a week to several times a day. They described three types of flashbacks; 1) perceptual, which were spontaneous recurrences of the visual effects of the acute LSD experience, 2) somatic, which were transient recurrences of altered body sensations which had been experienced during the acute experience, particularly numbness, parasthesias and pain, and 3) emotional, which were recurrences of the panic or fear they had experienced in the acute trip, and which could be so distressing the patient might feel suicidal. Despite many reports of the Flashback syndrome, it fell out of favor and has not been recognized as a medical entity. It appears that the third category, that of emotional flashbacks, has features akin to TPLSDS.

Little attention has been paid in the Psychiatric literature in the past three decades to pathology caused by LSD. One reason probably is that LSD fell into disfavor and there was less use and much less acute pathology after the 1970's. Unfortunately, in the past decade, there has been an increase in use of the drug, accompanied by an increase in acute toxic reactions.

In recent years several cases have been described of patients who were former users of LSD who became acutely ill after using a variety of medications. Aldurra and Crayton in 1993 reported a patient who developed visual disturbances 5 months after abstinence from LSD. He was admitted to a psychiatric unit because he felt suicidal, and stopped eating. He also had feelings of euphoria which were accompanied by geometrical visual hallucinations, blurred vision and black spots. He was treated with Risperidone, an antipsychotic, daily and became worse. He developed severe anxiety, became agitated and combative, said he felt crazier, and became more withdrawn and uncooperative. The patient was then switched to Olanzapine, with marked improvement.

Aldurra and Crayton focused on the harmful effect of Risperidone which they felt had made him much worse, and the beneficial effect of Olanzapine. They speculated on the relative binding or receptor site occupancy of Risperidone, Olanzapine, and LSD on particular neuronal receptor sites to explain the phenomena. Other authors have similarly speculated on the neuronal mechanism of action of Olanzapine and other medications in relation to LSD. This patient described by Aldurra and Crayton seems to be the first case of TPLSDS described in the literature, which their case report indicated was caused by the administration of

Risperidone. In 1996, Abraham and Mamen reported an exacerbation of "LSD-like panic" and visual symptoms caused by Risperidone in 3 patients who had been former LSD users.

There have also been reports of selective serotonin reuptake inhibitors (SSRIs) causing a recurrence of an LSD flashback syndrome. In 1994, Markel and Holmes reported on the exacerbation of the LSD flashback syndromes in two adolescents, former users of LSD, who were treated with antidepressants SSRIs. In 2007, Goldman, et al, described a 47-year-old patient who had a long history of depression and alcoholism, who "tripped out" after being prescribed several different antidepressants (SSRIs) after 2 decades of abstinence from LSD. The patient developed severe panic, rage, somatic symptoms and visual disturbances which he felt were similar to a bad trip on LSD. Both authors speculated on the mechanism of action of these phenomena, focusing on neuroreceptor physiology similarities of LSD and serotonin. It is difficult to avoid the conclusion that the cases described in this paragraph are either examples of TPLSDS or examples of reactivation of acute LSD toxicity by medications which have a synergistic effect with LSD. In any case, SSRIs are best avoided in TPLSDS.

There are no other pertinent references in the literature to the dangers of LSD.

Chapter 3

Treatment, Course of Illness, and Prognosis

As has been described in the above cases, the treatment of choice for TPLSDS is an antipsychotic medication. Olanzapine has been my drug of choice, and it has been extremely effective in producing full and complete remissions with manageable side effects. I chose it initially because it has been very effective for me in treating psychotic patients, and it had been particularly effective in treating acute toxic reactions to LSD. The patients I have treated with Olanzapine have found it helpful, and liked it. The treatment of these patients has been surprising in several ways – antipsychotic medication has usually been remarkably effective in relieving the symptoms, the required dosage has usually been remarkably low, and the medication has been required for longer than expected. An elaboration of these points follows.

Chapter 3

Patients usually reported that the first symptoms that were relieved were of the sleep disturbance and anxiety. With great relief, they reported that after only the first dose, they were able to fall asleep quickly, sleep soundly through the night, and had little or no racing thoughts or nightmares. As a result, they no longer felt exhausted the next day. There was also an immediate decrease in the severe anxiety and panic states and, within several days of being medicated, most patients felt and appeared to be much calmer. By the end of the first week, they were sleeping normally, felt calmer in general, and no longer had debilitating severe anxiety or panic states. They were elated and relieved that they were able to feel well.

Shortly thereafter, by the second week of treatment, improvement in ability to focus and concentrate was seen. Patients became able to sit and converse, to watch TV for a few minutes, and play a game. As intellectual functions and memory returned in the third week, patients became able to begin to read again gradually. Coping skills and ability to tolerate stress also returned. These functions improved gradually and steadily over the next month.

The improvement in the areas of emotional lability began more slowly, usually after two weeks of treatment, and continued gradually and steadily for weeks. Patients were relieved to no longer suddenly become overwhelmed with tears. They were surprised and relieved to no longer have anger surges which they had thought were fundamental and inherent in them. There usually was significant improvement in these areas of emotional lability within a month, with virtually complete resolution by the end of the second month.

Concomitant with these improvements, patients were better able to cope with stresses, both internal and external, and they felt more comfortable around people. Many patients after a month or two of these improvements began to consider a return to work or to school. I often found it remarkable that treatment was so effective and apparently complete. Usually the patient would respond so well to medication that within four to eight weeks the patient was in remission, free of symptoms, and appeared so calm, with such good affect, thought processes, and integration that he appeared to be normal.

I have found that the initial daily dose of Olanzapine required for effective therapy is usually 2.5 mgm., the smallest pill, given in a single bedtime dose. The bedtime dosage helped to treat the sleep disturbance more quickly and reduced the likelihood of daytime drowsiness or other side effects. This low dose of medication usually worked rapidly and effectively, as I just described above. When there is not sufficient improvement after a few days, the dose should be increased. I should add that patients who have a preexisting psychosis require larger doses, 5 to 10 mgm. of Olanzapine.

A minority of patients, immediately developed side effects, mainly feeling groggy and/or tired or nauseated. These symptoms were hard to tolerate and patients didn't know if they could continue the medication. When the dose was reduced properly, the side effects disappeared and the patients could resume the medication. I found it helpful to keep in mind that the initial dose was a guess, and the patient's somatic response helped us to find the correct dose, which was usually 50% or 25% of the original dose. For example, if I started a patient on 2.5 mgm. of Olanzapine, the smallest pill, and he felt groggy the next day, I would stop it until he no longer felt groggy, and then resume half the dose. If he became ill again, I would repeat the process. I found that in cases of sensitivity, one reduction in dosage usually sufficed, and I made two reductions in only a few cases. And in those cases the initial dose had generally been 5.0 mgm.

Most patients, after an initial period of weeks or months of stability on their original level of medication, experienced drowsiness, lethargy or weight gain as if oversaturated, and required a significant reduction in dosage. However, they needed to continue the medication even in low maintenance dosage for longer than expected. Most patients I have been able to follow have needed maintenance medication for at least 6 months, and many stayed on lowered doses of maintenance medication for several years. A typical example is a middle-aged woman who was treated initially with 2.5 mgm. of Olanzapine and by one year of treatment her dose had been cut in half. She continued in treatment for three more years, with further reductions and at termination was taking half a pill (1.25 mgm.) only twice a week. When she missed a dose, it was evidenced by increased anxiety, insomnia, and confusion. I found patients required doses I had previously considered to be homeopathic, in order to remain in remission. Even on these low doses, patients over a period of months often developed side effects, particularly drowsiness or weight gain, which indicated that a further reduction of medication was needed.

When patients felt well and reduced the medication too drastically or stopped it altogether, their symptoms returned, often with a vengeance, and they needed to resume the previous level of medication to go back into remission. If the medication was stopped abruptly, symptoms often recurred quickly. In some patients who reduced the medication gradually and then terminated it over a period of a month, the patients remained in remission for several weeks following termination before symptoms returned.

Other antipsychotics have been effective, but often not as fully as Olanzapine. Limited experiences with other anti-psychotics, e.g., Ziprazidone (Geodon), Aripiprazole (Abilify), and Quetiapine (Seroquel), thus far have brought significant, but usually incomplete improvement, and patients have felt and exhibited more full remissions when able

Chapter 3

to be switched to Olanzapine. The previous case discussions included several examples of treatment with alternate antipsychotics which produced considerable benefit and near-complete remissions. Nevertheless, Olanzapine seems to bring about a more complete relief from anxiety and anger, a more complete sense of calm and stability, and a greater improvement in cognitive and ego coping skills. There is a more complete improvement in fusion, resulting in a decrease in anger, and more complete improvement in the defensive, integrative and synthetic functions. Also, more patients receiving alternate antipsychotics, even in low doses, tended to have disturbing side effects more frequently than with Olanzapine. Some patients discontinued medications because of a skin rash, orthostatic hypotension, dizziness, nausea, or malaise, all of which were rare occurrences with Olanzapine in properly low doses.

I have had limited, but encouraging, experience with Thiothixene (Navane). Thiothixene has the benefit of being much less expensive than the relatively newer, atypical antipsychotics, such as Olanzapine, a significant factor for many State and County-supported patients. Although Thiothixene may not be quite as fully effective as Olanzapine, it seems to produce more complete remissions than the alternative antipsychotics, and with less side effects. The required dosage for effective treatment with alternate antipsychotics followed the model of Olanzapine; generally the smallest

THE POST-LSD SYNDROME

pill size available was an effective dose. However, some sensitive patients required only half of that smallest pill for effective initial treatment without side effects.

Anti-depressants and tranquilizers, which had been previously prescribed before the patients were referred to me, were seen to often have had a mild palliative effect on some of the symptoms, but did not bring about a full remission of any symptom, and sometimes caused negative reactions which led to discontinuation of the medications. Patients reported the anti-depressants primarily took the edge off of their anxiety, and may have helped them to fall asleep. There are also reports in the literature of specific adverse effects from some anti-depressants (SSRIs).

Prognosis with effective treatment appears to be excellent for remission of symptoms and a return to normal functioning. However, it is unclear as to how long treatment is necessary to cure the condition. It has been surprising that the patients seem to require the medication for prolonged periods of time, and some have not been able to discontinue medication even after several years. I have not been able to follow many patients for a long period of time, and more studies and data are needed to determine the curability of this condition. I have seen patients whose symptoms return if they discontinue or reduce their medication after one or two years of effective treatment. On the other hand, there are many patients who have gone into remission and then have been lost to follow-up, who may have had a cure.

Prognosis without effective treatment appears to be poor, as will be described in the cases that follow. These cases describe the continuing pathology these patients experience and their turning to alcoholism and other drugs.

There is also the issue of spontaneous remissions; many patients reported having had severe symptoms intermittently for many years, with spontaneous remissions, until the current illness caused sufficient distress to bring them into treatment. They reported periods of waxing and waning of symptoms, and the ability to tolerate or cope with the symptoms on their own to varying degrees, often for decades, before the symptoms became too severe to tolerate and they obtained treatment. Perhaps some patients experience a remission induced by treatment which may last for years, akin to the spontaneous remissions, which may not require maintenance medication, at least for some time.

CHAPTER 4

Alcoholism

When patients experience TPLSDS for years with only minimal benefit from ineffective medications, they become mentally and physically exhausted by the tetrad of symptoms, and are overwhelmed with discouragement, despair, helplessness and hopelessness. The reactive depression which most patients experience from the onset of the debilitating symptoms tends to intensify, adding to the distress. The natural progression for patients is to then turn to an addictive substance for relief.

The substance of choice for the majority of patients is alcohol, alone or in combination with marijuana, methamphetamines, cocaine, etc. They drink heavily, and gain palliative benefit by numbing themselves or drinking themselves into a stupor. The alcoholism further increases their inability to cope and to function, increases their helplessness and hopelessness, and increases their discouragement and anger with themselves. They

Chapter 4

state they are alcoholics, usually with guilt, shame, and hopelessness, and feel they cannot control the urge to drink. They are elated when effective treatment produces a remission of TPLSDS symptoms and they no longer feel a need to drink.

Case 5) Mr. E. was a 36 yr. old, married father of 3 who had developed a severe anxiety attack 6 months previously for which he was hospitalized and observed on a cardiac unit for 2 days. He had racing thoughts, terrible nightmares, constant anxiety, outbursts of anger, inability to concentrate, apprehension, and a feeling of doom. He'd had these symptoms intermittently since his early twenties, after he had taken LSD for a month, and had a terrible trip in which he became paranoid, terrified, acted crazy and got himself arrested. He said he never felt right after that, and then distressing acute symptoms developed, and he drank heavily and used drugs for over ten years to try to alleviate the symptoms. Two years before his consultation with me, he vowed to abstain from drugs and alcohol "for his family and his business", both of which he was in danger of losing. With great effort he had been successful for about a year, until the abrupt onset of his severe anxiety attacks six months previously.

On mental status, his affect was good and he showed no evidence of psychosis, though he had considerable anxiety, was discouraged and under great stress, and had trouble concentrating. He was started on Olanzapine, and had dramatic improvement. He slept better from the first night, his nightmares and racing thoughts dissipated in a few days, his anxiety improved rapidly within a week, and his ability to concentrate and cope became normal. On the medication he went into full remission within two months. He was elated that he felt able to function well in his daily life and wean off the alcohol without incident. After several months, he felt able to terminate, and said he would continue the medication, reducing it as needed.

Case 6) Mr. F. was 49-year old, self-proclaimed, life-long alcoholic who had been dry for three years after going through detoxification in a hospital, but recently had been experiencing increasing, severe anxiety which made him feel like drinking. He felt this was his life story, that he often felt extremely anxious for no reason, then became depressed, and then turned to drinking. He felt drinking had ruined his first marriage and his life, and he didn't want it to ruin his new marriage.

He had suffered a difficult childhood. He loved his father, a successful businessman and an alcoholic who often lost control of his temper, and then felt guilty and tried to make amends. The patient was smart, but unable to apply himself in school, and went to work for his father as a tradesman. His older brother, whom the father favored, worked in the front office with their father, was the heir-apparent, but was forced out after their father unexpectedly sold the business. His

Chapter 4

father died two years before Mr. F came to me, and he had unresolved grief because of his conflicting emotional issues regarding his father and his brother.

The patient said that in addition to his severe anxiety, he was depressed on and off for years, but anti-depressants didn't help much, and he typically became discouraged and turned to alcohol. He described difficulty concentrating, difficulty coping with stress and with feelings, and having surges of anger. He said he was struggling to avoid drinking again. In his second session, he told of his insomnia, racing thoughts at night, and terrible nightmares. He also said his anxiety at times reminded him of anxiety he experienced while using LSD in high school. We agreed on the diagnosis of TPLSDS, and started him on a low dose of Olanzapine.

He experienced immediate improvement. All symptoms waned rapidly; he felt enormous relief and within a week he said he no longer felt he needed to drink. He was able to abstain from alcohol and quickly weaned off of it. As he recovered, we gradually reduced the dose of his medicine. After a few months, he no longer felt troubled emotionally, and felt he had better coping skills than he had been aware of. He felt euphoria, and felt he no longer needed to be in regular therapy, but would continue his low dose of medication.

Case 7) Ms. G. was an intelligent, attractive, chronically depressed and unhappy 37-year old woman who was on medical marijuana for severe

THE POST-LSD SYNDROME

depression and anxiety, and had been alcoholic for years. She also used methamphetamines. Six months before I met her, she became violent, was arrested by the police and forced into a hospital program, where I eventually saw her. She had been diagnosed as Major Depressive Disorder and treated with an antidepressant. When that was ineffective, she was given Lithium, which also did not help.

In our first session, she told me that for months she had been experiencing severe anxiety, racing thoughts, insomnia, horrible nightmares, severe anger which was difficult to control, and increasing difficulty concentrating and coping. She said she had experienced them intermittently for years. Her attempts at self-medication with alcohol and marijuana had only taken the edge off of her anxiety. She worked intermittently as a waitress, a model, and an adult entertainer. She had never married, and had a series of boy friends. She had used LSD several times 15 years previously, until she had a bad trip which scared her. She said she became alcoholic after her bad trip.

She agreed to a trial of Olanzapine, and responded very well. Within one week she slept well, no longer experienced racing thoughts or nightmares, felt much calmer and better able to cope with stresses, and had much less anger. She was able to talk more effectively about her emotions and past traumas. She qualified for the Lilly Indigent Care Program and remained on the

Chapter 4

Olanzapine gratefully. She said she felt well, no longer needed hospitalization, and could function well. Over the next six months, she needed to cut her dose in half to avoid side effects, but found that if she discontinued the medication for several days, her symptoms returned.

Case 8) Mr. H. was a 52-year old man who was referred for evaluation of his treatment for Depression. He had been on antidepressants for twenty years, which he felt helped, but he was still depressed. He quickly reported he had been depressed for years, but had also experienced severe anxiety, severe insomnia with racing thoughts and terrible nightmares, irritability and anger outbursts, trouble coping and concentrating, and trouble controlling himself. He had used alcohol intermittently to alleviate the symptoms, but even heavy alcohol use combined with an antidepressant only worked partially.

He volunteered that at times he was reminded of feelings he had when he used LSD, even though he hadn't used LSD for 25 years. He said that at times he felt anxious, agitated, unstable, shaky, with a feeling of fear, paranoia, and doom, as he'd had when he was on LSD, but not as intensely. A low dose of an antipsychotic was administered, and brought about rapid and substantial relief of all symptoms. After two months, Mr. H. no longer felt depressed, felt the medicine was a miracle, and felt he would not need alcohol, or further treatment for the Depression.

Chapter 5

Depression

There are cases that are more challenging than others. The basic cases of TPLSDS are difficult enough of a diagnostic challenge. But, as the condition persists, and patients become more overtly depressed, but then fight against the depression with alcohol and other addictions which mask the clinical picture, the diagnosis is more difficult. In some cases there is a co-existing, internalized, emotional disturbance which manifests with depressive and behavioral symptoms. This disturbance requires therapy but is not accessible until TPLSDS is identified and treated.

Case 9) Mrs. I. was an attractive, artistic 49-year old former performer who was distraught and overwhelmed with anxiety and depression. For several years she had been going through a bitter divorce process which her vengeful, successful husband of 20 years was prolonging. She had been in twice-weekly psychotherapy for four

Chapter 5

years, was heavily medicated, and was addicted to Hydrocodone and Codeine.

She also was alcoholic, which she considered her main problem. She had received 3 DUIs, and had a pending court date to order imprisonment or long-term hospitalization. On mental status she was fairly intact, wanted to get well and no longer need addictive substances, She felt anxious and depressed, hypersensitive, hypervigilant, helpless, overwhelmed, and without direction. She wished she could get off of all addictive substances.

We agreed on twice-weekly psychotherapy, focusing on her grief over her divorce, her anxiety about being alone (an old issue for her), and her confusion and helplessness. A prime focus was helping her to protect herself, make good decisions, reduce her drinking, and wean her off of the Hydrocodone and Codeine.

She felt more clear-headed and less confused and distraught, but then began to experience more trouble sleeping, despite her sleeping pills. She soon developed terrible nightmares. They became vivid, bloody, intense and she awakened from them in a panic. In the dreams she was in terrible danger, often in a war situation threatened with death, and often fighting against being raped. She said when she awoke in terror, she felt as she had when she had a bad trip on LSD, and then remembered she had used LSD a few times in college and had some bad trips.

We then started Olanzapine with dramatic improvement. Her nightmares stopped, and she slept well. Her anxiety improved dramatically, and she was able to wean down more easily from her pain killers. She abstained from alcohol totally. She was more poised, self-contained, in control of herself and her emotions, and her judgement improved. She felt much better. We were able to convince the Court that it was best for her to remain in treatment rather than be forced into incarceration or long-term hospitalization, and she was placed on home monitoring with an electronic ankle device and probation for a year. She completed the program, during which she was free of alcohol, and was released from court supervision after a year.

She remained in therapy for several years. She weaned off of her addictive medications in a few months, made good progress in working on her emotional issues, and finally obtained her divorce. We gradually reduced her Olanzapine. Remarkably, after three years she was taking only 1.25 mgm (1/2 of the smallest pill) two to three times per week. When she tried to lower the dose too much, I could easily see her increased anxiety and decreased coping skills, and she could feel her symptoms exacerbating. As she progressed in therapy, she was free of drugs and alcohol, could cope and function well, and felt better about herself. She was able to establish new, relationships which appeared to be far superior to her previous ones, and she felt able to terminate her psychotherapy. She claimed she felt better than she ever had before, and was hopeful for her future.

Chapter 6

Addiction

There are many patients who are driven to addiction by the distressing symptoms of TPLSDS. Some are aware they suffer from incapacitating anxiety and mental exhaustion, but rarely realize the connection to their use of LSD.

Patients become addicted to the usual substances. As discussed above, alcohol is the substance most frequently abused by patients trying to quell the anxiety and distress caused by TPLSDS. Marijuana, amphetamines, and prescription medications are also frequently misused. Cocaine and heroin addictions are also seen, to a lesser extent. It is not unusual for a patient to present with multiple symptoms including addiction and depression, combined with the basic tetrad of symptoms of TPLSDS. Many patients use their addiction to deny awareness of the incapacitating anxiety and mental exhaustion, and avow they enjoy the addiction and will continue it. If they receive proper treatment, this attitude can change completely.

Case 11) Mr. K. was a self-proclaimed macho man, a 27 year old inmate with a history of heroin addiction, and aggressive, assaultive, violent behavior even in prison, where he was locked in maximum security. Although intelligent and academically successful in high school, he had wasted seven years of college by "living the good life, being macho" with alcohol, drugs, and womanizing, without completing a single academic course. His educated, loving parents, were distraught and helpless. He also had a violent, assaultive side, claimed to enjoy fighting, and developed a remarkable physique so he could look macho, and dominate in his fights. He had been arrested and imprisoned for possession and use of heroin, and claimed he would always be a heroin addict. He was referred to me for evaluation because of his anger, incorrigibility, and trouble sleeping. He seemed able to obtain drugs in prison.

He boasted of his wanton life style with pride and pleasure. He said he blew off his college classes because he enjoyed his playboy life style of heroin, women, and fighting. He slowly and reluctantly admitted to currently feeling very anxious at times, to having trouble concentrating, and to having trouble falling asleep. He protested repeatedly there was nothing wrong with him and he didn't want any medication. However, he liked talking, and agreed to continuing sessions. It took several

Chapter 6

months for him to reveal his racing thoughts at night, and his horrible nightmares. He clearly had surges of anger, but claimed that he wanted to be angry, and enjoyed it. He was afraid he'd become weak and vulnerable in his circle if he lost his angry edge.

He then admitted to having used LSD in high school, and then consented to a trial of Olanzapine. We were both surprised by how well he responded. His sleep disturbance and his anxiety improved and cleared rapidly. He was pleased by his gradually becoming able to concentrate, then able to read a few pages, and then able to read normally with comprehension and retention. He said he could see now that he had been unable to focus, read, and learn, and had been upset by that, and not known what to do. He had turned to alcohol and the drugs to escape from feeling helpless and depressed.

He thought now he could and would return to school successfully. His wanton life style had been a turning from "sour grapes" because of inability to perform academically. As he felt free of the racing thoughts and anxiety, he began to feel he would no longer need to use heroin, or anything else, as long as he could take his medication. He was then transferred to another prison, and was lost to follow-up.

Chapter 7

Suicide

It is striking that in this study of chronically distressed, dysfunctional, and ineffectively treated people there was only one grimly depressed, suicidal patient. Many patients expressed symptoms of depression, e.g. despondency, hopelessness, lack of energy, disinterest, etc., but they were not severely depressed or suicidal. Perhaps there is something inherent in TPLSDS which blocks affect and distracts the ego's attention that accounts for this. But whatever pathological effect LSD may have on the brain that lessens the danger of severe depression and suicide, this case is a stark reminder that suicide risk is a danger.

Case 12: Mr. L. was transferred from a maximum security psychiatric unit to our unlocked, minimum-security, psychiatric unit over the protests of our staff who feared we would be unable to keep him safe. He had successfully executed his grim plan to strangle himself, was found in coma

Chapter 7

by an unexpected visitor, and was maintained on life support for 48 hours in an Intensive Care Unit until he regained consciousness. When he awoke, he said he was sorry he was alive. He was transferred to a psychiatric maximum security unit, where he did not improve. He refused antidepressants and said he wished he had died. After three weeks he was transferred to our unit despite our opposition.

Mr. L. was a grim, joyless, 30-year-old, depressed man who was exhausted. He did not smile. He said he was sorry that he was alive; he had nothing to live for. He gave the impression that the failed suicide attempt had drained him, but he would soon have the energy to once again be suicidal. He said he was an alcoholic and had ruined his life because he couldn't stop drinking. His wife had left him "for the last time" a few months ago, but he had pleaded with her and she gave him one last chance. She stopped the divorce process, lifted the restraining order and hoped he would save their business and home. He said he loved her, but he was always letting her down. And now he had become alcoholic again, and she wanted to have nothing to do with him. She resumed the divorce process, restored the restraining order, and refused to see him or even talk to him. That was when he decided to kill himself. He did not blame her but he didn't want to live without her. She was a good wife for ten years, and he had been alcoholic for most of it.

I asked him why he drank, and he said he was alcoholic. I asked him if he liked drinking and he said not really. I asked him what happened when he didn't drink and he didn't know what I meant at first. Gradually he was able to say that when he did not drink he felt bad, nervous, scared, like something bad was going to happen. It was a very bad feeling. I said he was having severe anxiety and asked him if he had other bad feelings, and he described racing thoughts that kept him awake when he didn't drink.

I asked if he had other sleep problems, and he asked me how I knew. I told him I thought he may have a problem I'd seen before. He said sometimes he couldn't sleep because he got horrible nightmares and then he drank to stop them. He asked if I knew what caused this and I asked if he ever used LSD. He said he used it two or three times in high school but didn't really like it. I told him about TPLSDS in some detail, his mood lightened, and he said this might be him. He hoped so. We discussed medication and agreed to start an antipsychotic.

Mr. L. improved dramatically on the medication. He was less tense, more relaxed, and able to interact with others. He was able to sleep well. His grim, joyless mood cleared in a few days. He no longer felt a need to drink. He could see and feel that his mind was clearing, he was able to focus and concentrate better, and he was calmer. However, he still felt depressed about his wife who was continuing to refuse to see him. He continued to improve daily until his required discharge at two weeks. In his second week, his wife agreed to meet with me and

Chapter 7

him to discuss his condition and prognosis. She was surprised and pleased by the improvement in his mood and his thinking, she happily embraced him, told him she loved him, and hoped for the best. But she didn't want another disappointment for herself and the children. He said he wanted to get the business operating again and said he was feeling much better, and could probably return to it soon. She agreed to stop the divorce process and lift the restraining order. She said she would visit him daily, and he could visit his family daily after his discharge as long as he wasn't drinking. And then they would see what would happen.

Mr. L. completed his two weeks with continual improvement. At discharge, he wished our rules didn't prohibit follow-up, but said he'd continue the medicine as we'd discussed. His symptoms had greatly improved, and he had no need or desire. He still had a mild, lessening depression, with sadness and remorse over what he had put his family and himself through, but he was not grim or joyless, smiled, and was optimistic about his marriage, business, and life. He planned to live with a brother until his wife agreed to let him return, and he made arrangements to start up his business. There was no suicidal ideation or risk, and he said he was glad he did not die.

I wonder how many avoidable suicides have occurred in overwhelmed patients, as Mr. L. was, in whom TPLSDS was undiagnosed.

CHAPTER 8

Special Cases

Some patients are representative of a significant group of patients who have additional noteworthy pathology which dominates their presentation and their attitude about themselves which may obscure the recognition of The Post-LSD Syndrome initially.

1) PTSD

Case 13) Mr. M. was a 23-year old inmate who presented complaining resentfully that he had suffered a horrible childhood with unspeakable mental and physical abuses which had left him with terrible, painful memories and flashbacks. He had been told many times he had PTSD and needed treatment for it. To ease his pain, he had turned to drug and alcohol abuse, which had led to violations of the law and imprisonment. He was resentful, defensive and uncommunicative, asserting that talking only made him feel worse, and he did not

Chapter 8

want to discuss any symptoms because he felt that implied I didn't accept his PTSD. To him, the only thing that was important was that he had terrible memories and flashbacks almost constantly which made him feel horrible. He had been treated unsuccessfully with anti-depressants, and he was referred for evaluation of his medication.

As I worked with him for several weeks, he gradually described other symptoms —he had racing thoughts at night and could not fall asleep. When he did fall asleep, he slept very fitfully, and awoke at the slightest noise. He had terrible anxiety, and he had surges of anger. He could not sit still, could not focus, could not concentrate, could not watch TV or play a game, all, he felt, as a result of flashbacks from his PTSD. He then admitted to having horrible nightmares, which were vivid, intense, felt real, and were terrifying. After awakening, he often was disoriented and thought he was still in the nightmare. Sometimes the nightmares were not flashbacks of earlier trauma, but were bizarre scenes unconnected to anything from his past or present life. When I suggested he might be having some trouble because of his LSD usage, he bristled and took umbrage, again feeling I was trying to dismiss the PTSD. I said he could have both conditions, which would reenforce each other and make things worse for him.

He finally agreed to a trial of medication, and had a wonderful and gratifying improvement. After his first week on a low dose of an antipsychotic, he reported that he could not believe how much better he felt. His sleep had improved dramatically, and he now slept soundly without racing thoughts or nightmares. He felt rested and no longer was exhausted. His anxiety decreased, his anger surges diminished remarkably, and his affect improved over the next few weeks. He found himself smiling, felt well, started to enjoy things, and even felt happy at times. He said he felt better than he had ever felt before. He said the most amazing thing was that he still could remember the bad things he had experienced as a child, but he didn't think of them as much, and they didn't overwhelm him the way they had before. He said he didn't feel like the PTSD was the center of his life anymore. His mental condition became remarkably normal, with good intellect, ability to concentrate, good cognitive skills, and good affect. He still had some anxiety at times, but it was manageable. He began to feel optimistic about his future, and was grateful for the medication, but was then transferred to another prison.

2) Skin-head

Case 14) Mr. N. was a 50-year old lifer in a state prison who was a coarse, crude, angry white supremacist, a skin-head, who was referred because of his aggressive, violent outbursts directed at other inmates and at staff. He was set in his bigoted ways, was proud of his prejudiced views, and stated them loudly and boldly, even when outnumbered, causing concerns he could start a race riot or get himself

Chapter 8

killed. He was referred for a psychiatric evaluation, denied any problems or interest in therapy, and seemed to basically have a character disorder, with no suggestion of a psychosis. However, he did like talking more than we had expected, and did admit to having some anxiety and some difficulty sleeping. He agreed to take a mild anti-histamine to help him sleep. He agreed to monthly sessions, which I wanted for diagnostic and therapeutic purposes, and he seemed to get relief from them as he continued to vent his racial prejudices, paranoia, and other issues. Gradually, he talked of his past, admitted to heavy drug use, and then began to reveal his other symptoms.

He told of his racing thoughts, continual difficulty falling asleep, and increasing racial hatred. He had increasing concerns about his anger flaring up to the point he feared he would no longer be able to control himself. He feared he would become violent and lengthen his prison time. He then finally revealed his terrifying nightmares, and was ashamed and embarrassed that he could be so frightened. He admitted that sometimes, when he was anxious, he felt the way he had years ago when on acid. He finally agreed to a trial of medication, and felt great relief. His anxiety decreased quickly, his nightmares stopped, and his sleep improved within the first week. He was pleased and relieved. He was surprised when he "stopped feeling so hateful." After a few weeks, he told me with pride and amazement of walking with a friend, another white supremacist, who made a racial slur against another inmate. Mr. M. reported that he spontaneously told his friend that it wasn't necessary for him to talk that way, surprising himself and shocking his friend. He said he'd lost the racial hatred he'd thought was an integral part of him, and he felt better without it. He felt calmer, could think more clearly, and liked the way he now felt. He was then transferred to another prison.

3) Psychosis

Case 15) Mr. O. was a 32-year old dysfunctional man who was referred by a psychologist for medication for a Depressive Disorder with symptoms of depression and a sleep disturbance. He had had been in prison eight times, which constituted almost half of his life since he turned 18. After his original term, he then had seven violations, for trespassing, missing parole visits, testing positive for drugs, etc. He said he usually worked in a warehouse when he wasn't in prison, and drank a lot of alcohol because of anxiety and trouble sleeping. At times he was homeless. He had used methamphetamines for many years and some LSD, but discontinued them because he didn't like their effects. He had never been married, had 3 sons by 3 different women, but was barred by Court order from seeing them.

He was a tense, somber man who said he felt depressed, hadn't been able to sleep, had developed

Chapter 8

racing thoughts, felt sluggish and unable to think, and had increasing difficulty concentrating. He also had recently developed severe, intense, horrible nightmares from which he awoke in terror. For the past two months he had again felt increasingly unable to tolerate stress, had anger surges, and often felt like blowing up. He was extremely worried because he said he "could get angry in a flash" so suddenly that it caught him by surprise and felt difficult to control. He had experienced these symptoms intermittently and to varying degrees for years.

He had voluntarily talked with a psychiatrist for 2 years in a clinic in recent years, and had been evaluated by mental health personnel repeatedly in prison, but had never been diagnosed as having significant pathology, nor taken any medicine. He admitted that for the past year he'd heard voices calling his name during the day, as he'd heard intermittently over the years, but had never previously revealed that to anyone. Clinically, Mr. O. evidenced flattening of affect, concrete thinking, and autistic withdrawal, which were obscured by the symptoms of TPLSDS. We agreed to medicate him with an antipsychotic and he responded well. After one week, he reported he was sleeping well for 4-5 hours a night, had less racing thought, felt calmer, less anxious, less irritable, less stressed out and the voices and nightmares had stopped. He said at times he felt happy.

It was clear TPLSDS had gone into remission. His affect had improved and he smiled at times. However, he continued to manifest a degree of flattening of affect, concrete thinking, a degree of autistic withdrawal, and paranoid ideation which indicated a chronic, psychotic process which also was now largely into remission. We increased his medication, and his improvement continued over the next few weeks. He became optimistic about being able to have a better life with the help of his medication, as he was able to feel he had better judgement and self-control. It appeared that both TPLSDS and Psychosis were in remission.

Chapter 9

Barry

Barry was 16 years old when he was referred to me over 25 years ago. He was a pleasant, friendly, bright, outgoing, troubled and dysfunctional youngster whom his parents were very fond of, indulged, and referred to as a "nice boy" despite his delinquent and incorrigible behavior. He truanted from school, underperformed academically, disobeyed them constantly, used marijuana habitually, and stole from them. He also had severe anxiety attacks, had trouble sleeping unless he used marijuana, and was unhappy with himself. I felt he had an emotional disorder and had no concept of TPLSDS at that time.

Barry related to me well, agreed he was neither happy with himself nor in control of himself, and agreed to psychotherapy twice weekly. He came faithfully, worked in earnest on his feelings and his issues, and made some progress over his first year in therapy. He fought with himself and his parents less, felt better, became less anxious, stopped truanting, and decided to stop using drugs and alcohol. He discontinued usage of drugs and alcohol fairly easily except for marijuana. As he reduced the marijuana, he had increasing difficulty sleeping. But he persisted, ended his marijuana use, but then became increasingly anxious, unable to sleep, developed horrible nightmares, and became frantic as he was getting only a few hours of sleep a night. He said his mind would not shut off. He felt desperate, felt he needed to talk to me every day, was afraid he would slip back to using marijuana, and asked to be hospitalized. I complied, and he was hospitalized for a month. While he was hospitalized, we met four times a week in 50 minute sessions, and he strove to talk about his issues and feelings. He worked hard, but there was little benefit.

Upon his discharge, he couldn't sleep, and in desperation smoked marijuana again for several nights. At his next session, he told me he'd smoked marijuana, it had relaxed him and enabled him to sleep for 2 nights, but then he developed a bad trip which reminded him of the last time he'd used LSD several years previously. He had again become confused, anxious, paranoid, saw the walls moving, had visual tracings, and felt terrible. Even though he hadn't had any marijuana for over 24 hours, he still was in a panic and saw the visual tracings constantly. He was convinced he hadn't had any LSD on this occasion, but that the marijuana had triggered off an acute LSD reaction. Because of his distress, symptoms of drug toxicity, and my concern about his LSD exposure, I treated him with Thioridazine, an anti-psychotic medication which I had found helpful in treating acute psychosis and acute LSD psychotic reactions.

Barry responded very well to the relatively low dose of Thioridazine. He slept well from the first night he took it. His acute, toxic symptoms cleared quickly. He was no longer in a panic, and his mind cleared. He no longer had visual distortions, tracings, nightmares, or racing thoughts. We found that he needed to stay on the medication after his symptoms subsided, or the insomnia and the anxiety would return. As he took the medication, we saw improvement in his state of mind; he was less anxious, less prone to become overwhelmed by feelings and anxiety, and was able to concentrate and focus better. He seemed to be more integrated and get more benefit from his therapy. At no time was there ever an indication he was psychotic. He continued in his therapy twice weekly for several years and we were able to work more effectively on his numerous issues and conflicts which ranged from adolescent, to familial, to neurotic issues. He continued Thioridazine in smaller doses for over a year, reduced it from daily to several times a week, until he concluded therapy and moved out of state to go to college.

I concluded that he had an Adolescent Adjustment Reaction, complicated by LSD use with subsequent LSD toxic reactions. However, the dose of Thioridazine he required acutely was unusually low, as was his need to continue the medicine for so long in order to prevent a return of symptoms. In retrospect now, I think Barry had an Adolescent Adjustment Reaction complicated by TPLSDS which was his primary pathology.. His psychotherapy was helpful, but his anti-psychotic medication was essential and curative.

Bibliography

1. Abraham, H. and Aldridge, A.: Adverse Consequences of LSD. Addiction. 1993. 88:1327-1334.
2. Abraham, H. and Mamen, A.: LSD-Like Panic From Risperidone in Post-LSD Visual Disorder. J. Clin Psychopharm. 1996. 16:238-241.
3. Aldura, G. and Crayton, J.: Improvement of Hallucinogen-Induced Persistent Perception Disorder: Case Report. J. Clin. Psychopharm. 2001. 21:343-344.
4. Brewer, Robt.: Chronic Pathology Caused by Methamphetamine. Unpublished. Personal Communication.
5. Cohen, S.: LSD: Side Effects and Complications. J. Nerv. Ment. Dis. 1960. 130:20-40.
6. Idem: Psychosomatics: A Classification of LSD Complications. 1966. 7:182-186.
7. Cohen, S. and Ditman, K.S.: Prolonged Adverse Reactions to LSD. Arch. Gen. Psych. 1963. 475-480.
8. Cooper, H.A.: Lancet, 1:1078, 1955
9. Eveloff, H.: The LSD Syndrome. Cal. Med. J. 1968. 109-368-373.
10. Frosch, W.A., Robbins, E.S., and Stern, M.: Untoward Reactions to LSD. 1965. NEJM, 273:1235-1239.

11. Goldman, S., Galarneau, D., and Friedman, R.: New Onset LSD Flashback Syndrome Triggered by SSRI. Ochsner J. 2007. 7:37-39.
12. Hoffman, Albert:: LSD: My Problem Child. 1980
13. Leary, T.: Introduction in LSD, edited by D. Solomon, G.P. Putnam's Sons, New York 1964
14. Ludwig, A.M. and Levine, J.: JAMA, 191:92, 1965
15. Markel, H., Holmes, R., Domino, E.: LSD Flashback Syndrome Exacerbated by SSRIs in Adolescents. J. Ped. 1994. 125:817-819.
16. Rosenthal, S. Persistent Hallucinosis Following Following Repeated Administration of Hallucinogenic Drugs. Amer. J. Psychiat. 1964. 121:238-244.
17. Savage, C.: J. Nerv. Ment. Dis.: 125:434, 1957
18. Shick, F. and Smith, D.: Analysis Of The LSD Flashback. J. of Psychedelic Drugs. 1970. 1:13-19.
19. Smart, A. and Bateman, B.: Unfavorable Reactions to LSD. Canadian Med. J. 1967. 97:1214-1221.
20. Ungerleider, J., Fisher, D., and Fuller, M. The Dangers of LSD. J.A.M.A. 1966. 197:389-392.
21. Vardy, M. and Kay, S.: LSD Psychosis or LSD-Induced Schizophrenia?. Arch. Gen.Psych. 1983.

Author Biography

Dr. Roth was born and raised in East Cleveland, Ohio. He graduated from Adelbert College and the Medical School of Western Reserve U. He then trained in Pediatrics at Jacobi Hospital in the Bronx, New York, and was drafted from his Residency to serve in the USAF during the Cuban Missile Crisis. He served in Spain and Morocco in the Strategic Air Command (SAC) as a Pediatrician. Upon his discharge, he returned to Cleveland as a Resident in Psychiatry and then a Fellow in Child Psychiatry at University Hospitals of Cleveland. After a year as Child Psychiatric Consultant to B&C Hospital, he became Director of the Child Psychiatry OPD for six years. He became a diplomate of the American Board of Psychiatry and Neurology and then of the American Board of Child Psychiatry. He went into full time private practice in 1975, and was a Consultant for many years to Cuyahoga County at Juvenile Court, Metzenbaum Children's Center, and Hudson Boy's School. He was also a Treatment Team Leader at Bellefaire Residential Treatment Center. His main focus has been direct clinical practice. He graduated from the Cleveland Psychoanalytic Institute in both Adult and Child Psychoanalysis, and has engaged in the full time practice of Adult, Child and Adolescent Psychiatry and Adult and Child Psychoanalysis for over 30 years.

After relocating to Palm Desert in southern California in 1997, Dr. Roth began to become aware of the patients who became the subject of this book. Working in his private practice and as a part-time Psychiatrist for Riverside County Mental Health and then for the California Department of Corrections and Rehabilitation at Chuckawalla Valley State Prison, he came in contact with patients who presented a different pathology than he had noted previously. He became increasingly aware of the existence of this condition, The Post-LSD Syndrome, and its surprising lack of recognition. He then researched the literature intensively, only to find a total lack of recognition in the literature. Because of the severity of the disturbance, its attendant suffering, and the relative treatability of the condition, Dr. Roth felt The Post-LSD Syndrome should be brought to public attention.

The website for Dr. Roth and this book can be accessed at edwinrothmd.com or at the post-lsdsyndrome.com.

www.ingramcontent.com/pod-product-compliance
Lightning Source LLC
Chambersburg PA
CBHW021017180526
45163CB00005B/2001